The Magic of Radishes

To Cure and to Heal

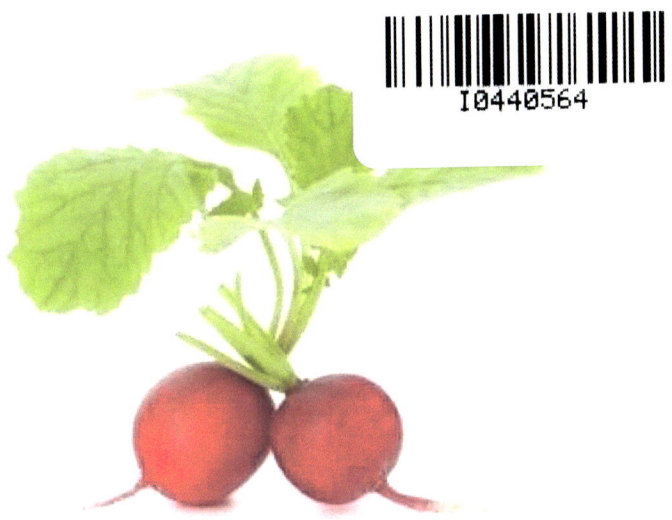

I0440564

Dueep Jyot Singh

Natural Remedy Series

Mendon Cottage Books

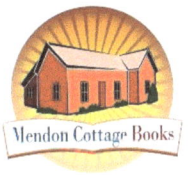

JD-Biz Publishing

Disclaimer

The information is this book is provided for informational purposes only. It is not intended to be used and medical advice or a substitute for proper medical treatment by a qualified health care provider. The information is believed to be accurate as presented based on research by the author.

The contents have not been evaluated by the U.S. Food and Drug Administration or any other Government or Health Organization and the contents in this book are not to be used to treat cure or prevent disease.

The author or publisher is not responsible for the use or safety of any diet, procedure or treatment mentioned in this book. The author or publisher is not responsible for errors or omissions that may exist.

Warning

The Book is for informational purposes only and before taking on any diet, treatment or medical procedure, it is recommended to consult with your primary health care provider.

Our books are available at

1. Amazon.com
2. Barnes and Noble
3. Itunes
4. Kobo
5. Smashwords
6. Google Play Books

Table of Contents

Introduction – Knowing More about Radishes

I was once being shown around the organic farm of a friend of mine, and I noticed him giving me rather funny looks. "You have never been around an organic farm before, have you? Or it is possible that you have not lived in this area, have you." Naturally, I had to ask him what made him say that, because I was used to going around organic farms, once being an organic gardener myself. He said that any native of that particular area would immediately pounce upon a radish growing in the fields, and pull it out – without waiting for an invitation from the owner – dip it into the nearest water source, and sink his teeth into it.

When in Rome do as the Romans do. I did so. And thus I enjoyed the crisp natural sweetish taste of this taproot, Raphanus sativus, which has been the mainstay of so many civilizations since prehistoric times.

The Romans could not do without the radish. In fact, it was eaten raw, cooked, boiled, made into salads, and not only the taproot, but even the leaves were finished by those people who enjoyed good food.

The ancient Greeks and Romans used to make a paste of radish and onions with dried fish and eat it with every meal. In fact Apicius has spoken about radishes, best eaten with pepper in "his Art Of Cooking in Imperial Rome." So I would not be surprised if the ubiquitous fish sauce, used to liquefy and spice dishes, and known as garum was not also added to dishes with another sharp flavoring agent – radish.

One is grateful that radishes are available all over the world, but whether people use them for their own benefit as much as they should, is debatable. That is because many people think that radishes like onions and garlic have a distinctive odor. That is why, at parties or at get-togethers, they are just served as salad helpings, accompanied with onion slices and tomatoes.

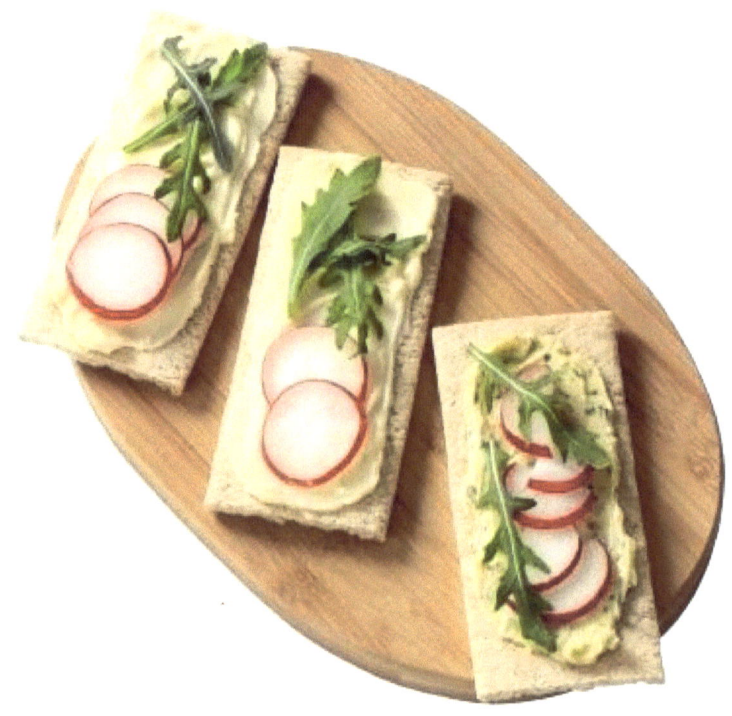

Radishes on buttered bread

The radish got its generic name Raphanus from the Greek word meaning "that which appears quickly". That is because the farmers knew that they just had to sow these radish sprouts and seedlings and they would be ready to harvest really fast. It is believed that the radish originated in West Asia. Nowadays, the best well-known radish producing countries in the world are South Africa, China, – where it was cultivated more than 3000 years ago – and Indonesia, India, Malaysia and other hot climates.

Even though they are no apparently readily available historical and archaeological document records in the West, talking about the cultivation of the radish in ancient Greece and Rome, yet, this cultivated plant was an integral part of Eastern cuisine and medicine, including Chinese medicine, Korean medicine and Indian medicine for millenniums.

Radish was fermented and used as a relish, – kimchi – for millenniums in Korea. Allied radish dishes are also part of Chinese cuisine.

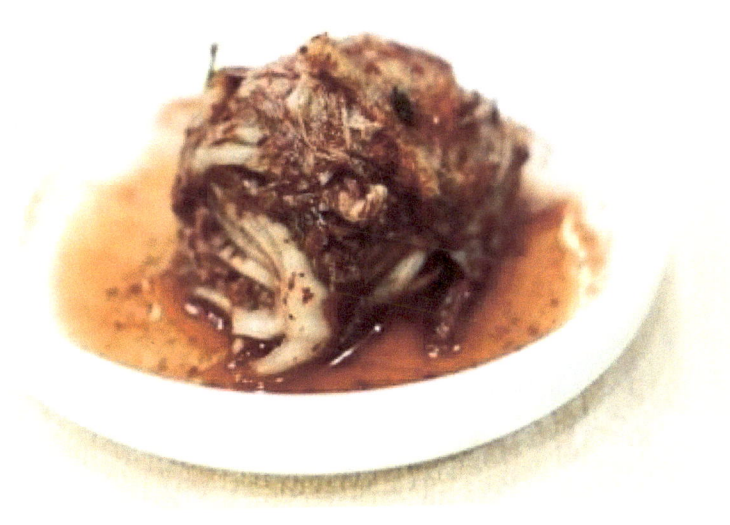

This is how radish kimchi should look

How to Grow Radishes

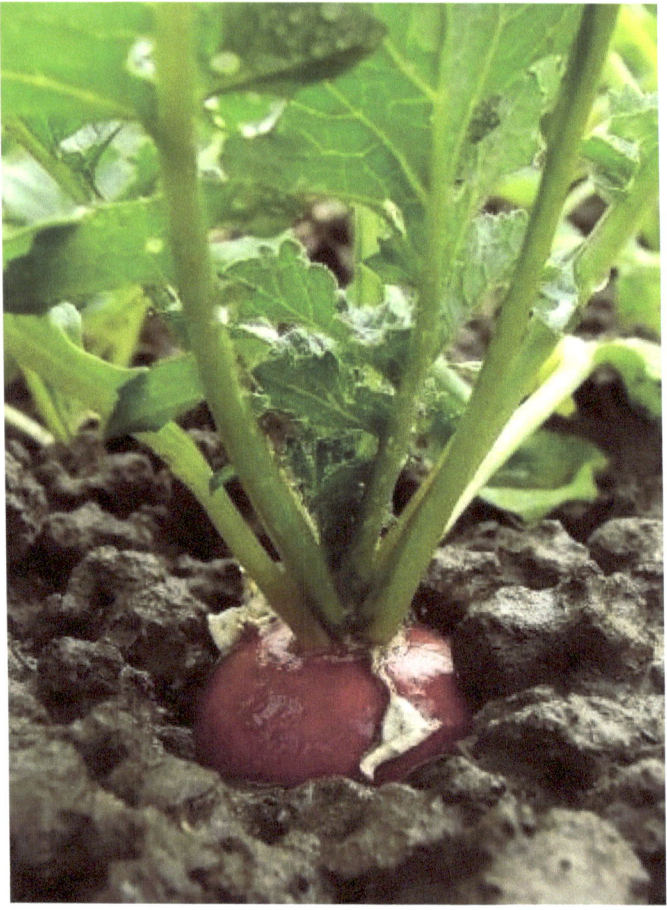

If you want a rich radish harvest this year, look for different varieties and choose the one which best suits your requirements. Radishes can be grown all through the year, depending on the hybrid variety. Nevertheless, if you want the spring harvest from a winter sowing, you can choose a slow maturing variety like *French Breakfast*.

Growing radish plants is best done in areas which have plenty of sun. Radishes love soil, which is loamy and sandy with an excellent drainage system. In North America, radishes can be sown from early spring to June and from October – January, depending on the variety. However, in Japan, China, and India, they are available all year around, because they are planted in areas which are not subject to heavy snow falls in winter.

I would advise you not to plant radishes in the summer, because then the growing is lessened. But spring planting and autumn planting is excellent. So if you are a first-time gardener, try planting radishes.

You can either sow the seeds directly in a well fertilized and moist bed. In greenhouses, these seeds are planted at the depth of 1 ½ inches – for the small radish varieties and up to 4 inches for the large variety – and 2 inches apart. These are normally planted in rows which are 12 inches – 18 inches apart.

If you crowd the seedlings, while planting, they are definitely not to grow well. Because even though they are a taproot vegetable, they want some space, both up and down, where they can spread and flourish.

In the East, farmers normally put in crops for a three-year rotation. That is, so that they can get an uninterrupted harvest of these fast-growing plants. They keep planting every two weeks. By the time these plants have grown, there is going to be another crop ready for harvesting.

Try planting in early fall. You are going to get a harvest before the winter sets in.

Harvesting Your Radishes

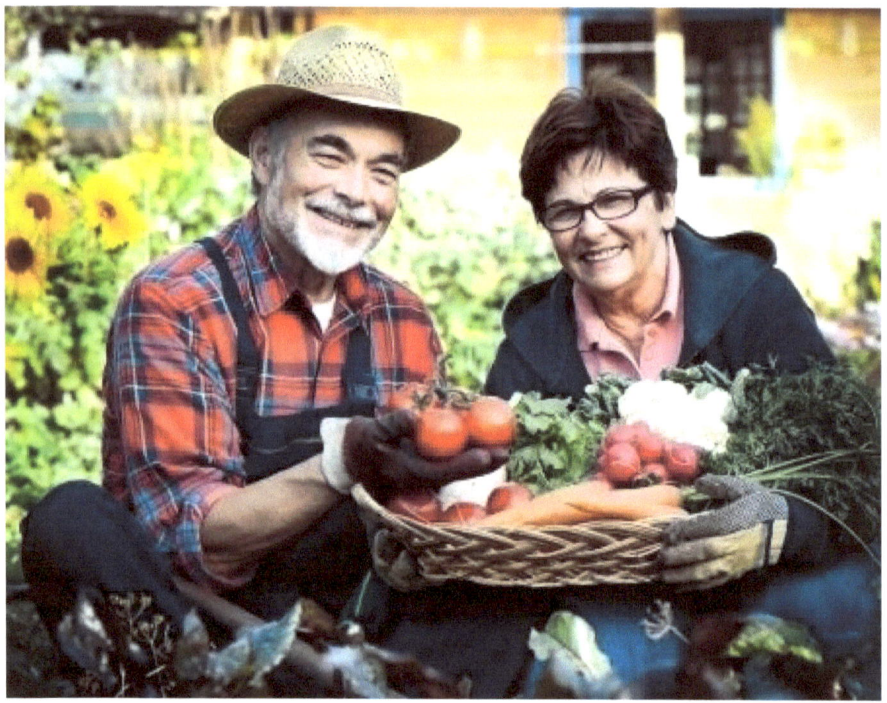

What an achievement a harvest of your own farm grown or homegrown vegetables included radishes is!

Your radishes are going to be ready to harvest within three weeks of sowing. Once they have matured, remember to harvest them, because if they stay too long in the earth, they are going to turn bitter in taste. A freshly harvested radish has a sweet/sharp taste with no taste of bitterness.

Remove the greens and store them separately. These greens are going to start turning yellow, after three days. So use them in salads. As soon as you harvest the radish crop, cut off the tops. Wash and then dry the radishes and then place them in plastic bags. Store them in the refrigerator immediately. Like carrots, they are definitely not going to keep their crispness if they are left unpackaged in the refrigerator for more than three days. They are going to keep for up to two months, in the refrigerator at 0°C.

Here is an amazing historical fact. Some archaeologists found radish seeds from digs in Greece and sowed them. And 4 plants came up! Well, seeds are very hardy, because many of us budding archaeologists know the story about those lotus seeds, buried more than 2000 years ago, in one of the Pharaoh's lily ponds, which germinated in a greenhouse in the 21st century, under controlled conditions. This is one of the most wonderful things about nature.

By the way, the hanging Gardens of Babylon were not made by Nebuchadnezzar,- as was said by a historian in 1BC – who mixed his names of kings, and was believed by the rest of the world,- but by the Assyrian king Sennacherib in Nineveh about 300 miles away from Babylon. So just imagine the world of now extinct plants and animals, which are just waiting to be unearthed. Perhaps we are going to find radishes, there.

Sad to say, all those miraculous plants and vegetables, buried under the ashes of Herculaneum and Pompeii were totally cooked, so there is no question of us eating vegetables, which were cultivated millenniums ago from those seeds.

Soils

Radishes can grow in any soil, except unless you intend to sow them in one particular season. Like if you are looking to sow them in the winter or in the spring, you may want the soil to be sandy. Any soil, which solidifies in the winter, is definitely not suitable for taproot growth.

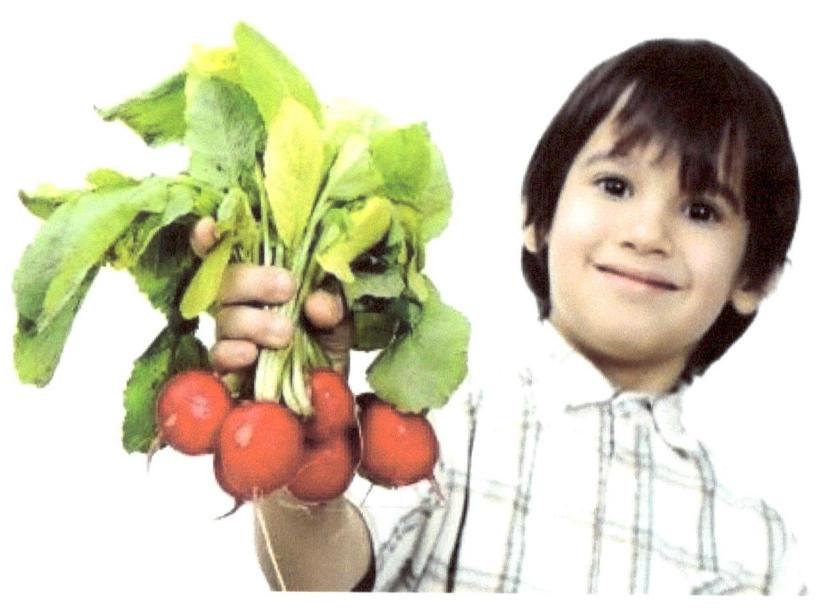

Radishes are an excellent plant choice to encourage children in gardening. In fact, my brother asked his kids to choose their own garden patch and provided them with radish seeds. They were extremely thrilled to see those seedlings coming up within three days, and they became so possessive about their radishes, that they would not have them eaten! So now those radishes are preserved in a plastic bag to be trotted out to the admiring adults, who come to see what is cooking in an organic kitchen garden!

Summer Radishes

If you are planting radishes in the summer, look for varieties which are going to germinate within three days. Yes, there are some varieties like *April Cross* and *Cherry Belle,* which are going to mature within a month.

Here are some spring varieties as well as summer varieties – *Champion, Bunny Tail, Plum Purple* and *Red King.* If you ask for an *Easter Egg* combination you are going to get a mixture of a number of seed colors, from white to red to purple!

Winter Radishes

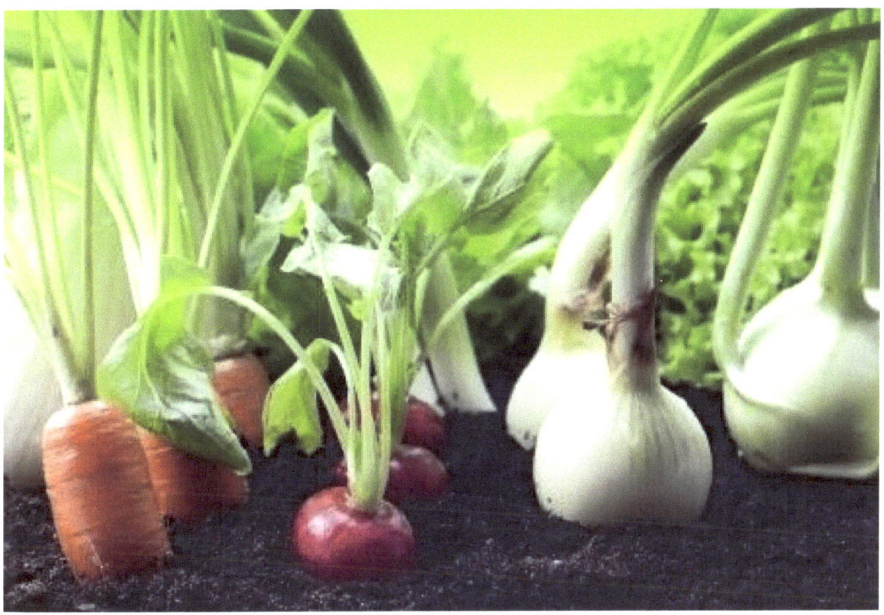

Try growing onions and carrots along with radishes

The Japanese and Korean as well as the Indian varieties, especially those cultivated in Asia belong to this group. *Daikon* is the most popular variety here. It is also called *Chinese Radish, Japanese Radish* and Indian radish or *Mooli*.

If you want something really hot, try the Japanese *Sakurajima daikon.* It is the grand pappy of all the Sumo radishes, growing up to 10 pounds. We could just buy one of these sumos and subsist throughout the winter on that one vegetable. A Japanese friend Katsuko,told me that she had won a kitchen garden prize for her Sakurajima , which went up to 30 kgs, - *Woweee-* because she forgot to harvest one particular plant and allowed it to ripen underground. And because it had plenty of time to garner unto itself the nutrients of a harvested radish field, it grew and it grew and it grew just like pumpkins do in fairytale stories.

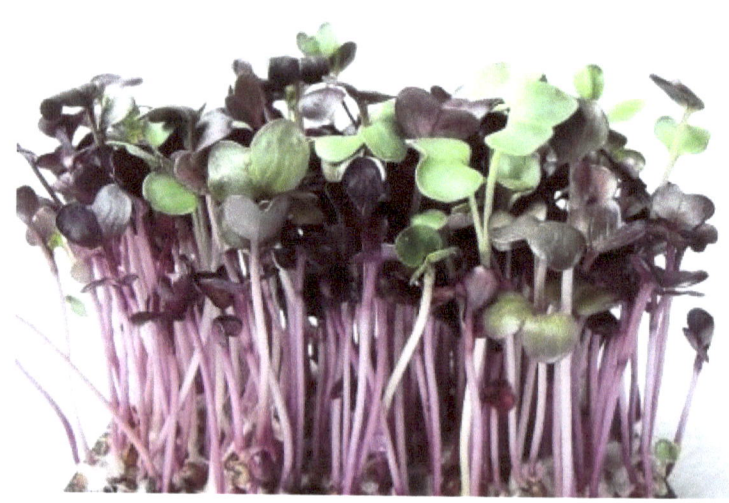

Red radish sprouts

If your radishes have been allowed to seed, collect them and use some of them in salads. They are spicy and tasty. In fact, the rat tailed radish is grown for its seats, instead of its taproot. If you are in Germany, and want something crunchy to eat, it is possible that you will be given the seeds of *München Bier* radish, to munch with your beer.

Radishes are extremely rich in vitamin C and potassium. That is why I overheard someone suffering from cramps in the legs to eat more radishes, because that would cure him. He was supposedly suffering from a potassium deficiency, which could also be cured by eating two bananas per day, continuously for a month. But radishes are definitely more effective and better.

Radish sprouts are also delicious to eat, just like mung bean sprouts.

Radishes in Cuisine

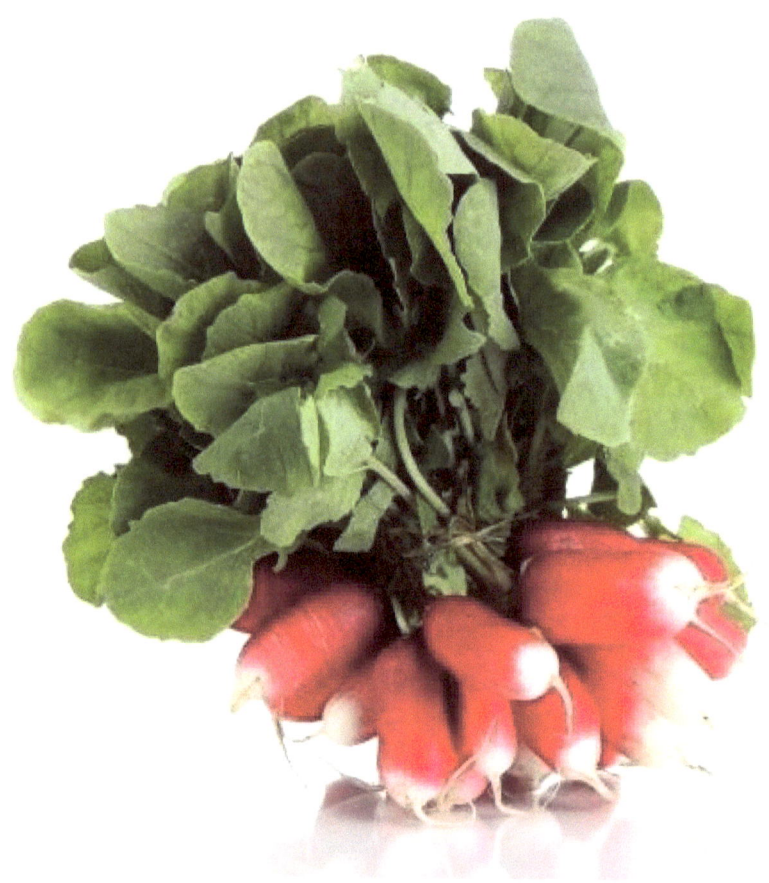

Try using radish leaves as salad greens

If you are using fresh pink or red radishes, you do not need to peel them. Just chop them up into small pieces, wash and eat raw. You can also add salt and pepper and munch them with bread and butter. French cooks normally make radish sauces with Roquefort cheese, with huge sprinklings of red cayenne pepper. Also, these red radishes are extremely good-looking in salads with onions and tossed with olive oil or salad oil, vinegar, as well as a little bit of honey to soften up the sharp taste. Radishes can be cooked glazed or creamed, just like you do carrots and turnips.

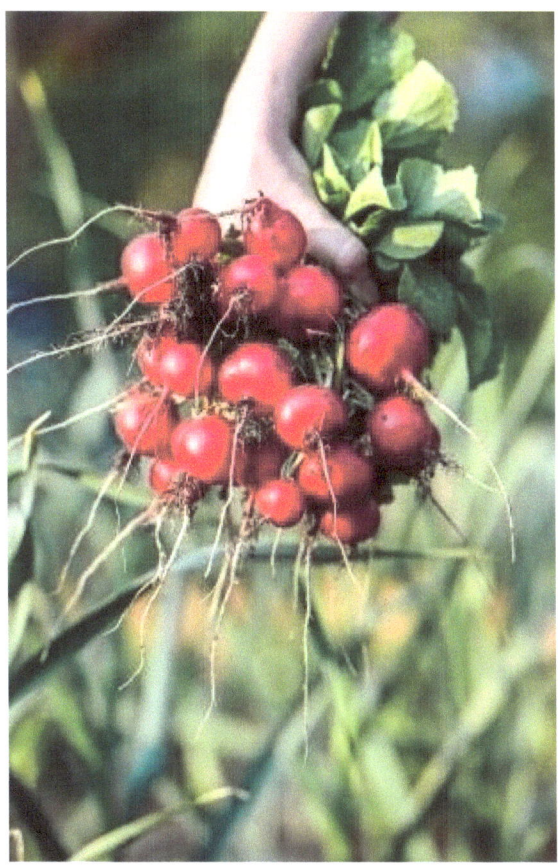

Fresh green radish tops can be washed and cooked with potatoes in a soup or in a potage. Like I said before they last for three days, before turning yellow.

The French and Italians love black radishes, because they are so very sharp tasting. Red and pink radishes are milder in taste. You just slice up the black radishes, salt and season them according to your taste and make them into sauces, or just add them to yogurt with onions and shallots. Try the vinegar, honey and radish combination. Delicious when eaten with bread, butter and roasted meat.

Wheat Radish Salad with Yogurt

This is a very healthy salad served and enough for 12 glasses. Preparation time is 25 minutes and cooking time is 10 minutes. Easy to make and nice to eat.

Ingredients needed are –

150 g of precooked wheat
Half a cucumber.
Two tomatoes – try the Californian variety or the Roman variety.
Half a bunch of radishes-four will do just fine.
150 g of fresh yogurt.
2 tablespoons balsamic vinegar
Juice of one lemon
2 tablespoons olive oil
Half a bouquet of chives
Salt and pepper, and any other seasoning to taste.
Let some salted water boil in the casserole and then allow the precooked wheat to cook in it for 10 more minutes. Drain and then pass the wheat under running water so that the cooking process is stopped. Put aside.

Wash the vegetables, then chop up the cucumber and the tomatoes into 1 cm in diameter pieces. You can also chop up the radishes and their tops in small slices.

Put the salad in the salad bowl, mix the wheat with the cucumber and the tomatoes, the slices of radish, the lemon juice and the olive oil. Season according to taste with salt and pepper, and then "scissor" the chives right on top of the salad.

 In another bowl, mix the yogurt with the balsamic vinegar, salt and pepper. Place this mixture right at the bottom of the glasses.

Now place the radish wheat mixture right on top of the yogurt, and serve chilled.

Apple Sauce with Horse Radish

Preserved Horseradish is easily found on your supermarket shelves.

This was a favorite dish in British times, especially with Anglo-Indian army officers, who wanted something delicious to eat with cold poultry and roasted meat. Horseradish and roasted meat is a common combination in British cuisine, but the Anglo Indian version is applesauce and horseradish! By the way, this particular combination is Yugoslavian in origin. From Yugoslavia to the Delhi gymkhana club – it is a small world!

2 ounces of horseradish, grated

4 ounces of yogurt.

4 ounces of cream.

4 ounces of crisp eating apple grated

Honey to taste.

Add all these ingredients to the horseradish one at a time. Mix well, and chill overnight, because the taste is going to improve, if you eat it. One day after you have made it, with slices of cold meat, poultry, turkey, or anything else.

Thai Meat Salad With Radish

Six pieces of already roasted meat. You can either use chopped meat pieces, or chicken breast.

You are going to marinate the roasted meat in two cloves of garlic, one piece of crushed ginger, three pinches of salt for seasoning and 1 tablespoon full of olive oil. Put the meat pieces in this marinade and mix very well with your hands.

The salad is going to consist of 12 lettuce leaves, two small cucumbers, one bunch coriander leaves, washed, 12 radishes and some mint leaves for garnishing.

The vinaigrette is going to consist of 4 teaspoons full of mixed fish sauce, also known as **Nuoc Mam cham,** the juice of one unripe lemon, one teaspoonful of sugar and half a teaspoonful of red chili peppers powder.

http://www.youtube.com/watch?v=6fUu0l6_60U – how you make a fish sauce. This is a dipping sauce, which is very popular among the Vietnamese and the Thais.

This is what is going to add the exotic quality to your radish, meat and fish salad.

The vinaigrette is prepared by mixing up the sugar, the fish sauce, the pepper and the sugar.

Place the lettuce leaves on four plates or on one large serving salad plate.

Chop the cucumber into small bits and spread them all over the lettuce leaves. Do the same thing for the radishes cut in slivers and spread them on the salad. Add the mint and the coriander, chopped fine, or scissored all over the salad, vegetables.

Heat a frying pan or a skillet and then re-cook the roasted meat, along with its marinade from all sides, keeping the meat pink and juicy.

Place the pieces of meat on a chopping board. Allow to cool for two minutes before slicing.

Divide the meat portions on all the plates or on the large serving plate, and then sprinkle the salad with the vinaigrette.

Serve this salad immediately.

Kimchi-or Fermented Radish/Cabbage

Kimchi is getting to be known as one of the most popular of traditional and ancient Korean dishes, in the West. Thanks to its healthy ingredients, subtle flavorings, sour, sweet and spicy taste, the national dish of Korea is now being presented here, for your good health.

Early Kimchi was made up of cabbage and meat stock in ancient times. Red peppers were not introduced until the 14 century by the Japanese, and soon, they became an integral part of the Kimchi, to give it a hot flavor. There is a museum in Seoul dedicated totally to kimchi, which has 187 current as well as historic varieties versions and recipes of this dish.

The ingredients are one Chinese cabbage, but you can also use four radishes or turnips. This is going to be mixed Kimchi.

One small clove of garlic, as well as a tiny piece of chopped ginger, – the same quantity as the garlic.

One Apple -cooking

4 tablespoons full of red chili powder – it is going to be hot!

2 tablespoons full of sugar

Chop the Chinese cabbage, radish and turnips, into small squares.

When you have finished chopping up all the vegetables, place all of these pieces in a glass pickle container. Add salt, so that all the liquid can get absorbed but do not add so much of the salt so that this recipe becomes thoroughly inedible.

You may want to use your own estimate. Consider yourself making pickles.

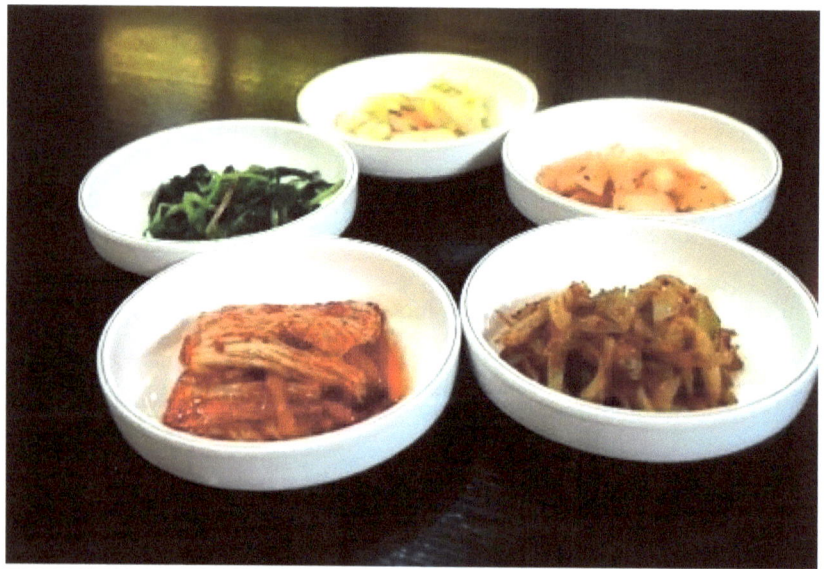

Traditional Korean kimchi made up of different vegetables

Cover the container with its air tight lid. Place in the sun in a shady place. Kimchi is ready within one day, in summer, but it needs three days of winter sun, depending on the level of the humidity and the temperature.

The radish and the cabbage is going to dry out within a couple of days, thanks to the salt. Now grate the Apple, garlic and ginger and place it in a container.

The ingredients, which are going to be using now are the garlic, ginger, Apple, red chili powder, salt and sugar.

Boil a glass of water, and pour it in the bowl, in which you have put the salt, red chili powder and the sugar. This water is excellent for mixing all these items. Now add the grated mixture to this sugar, chili powder mixture.

Add the sun dried and salted cabbage/radish a little by little.to this liquid, stirring all the while. This kimchi can be eaten now, but I would suggest allowing it to ferment a little more for some days. It is going to be even tastier.

Kimchi is delicious eaten fresh or eaten preserved. Kimchi is normally served with rice and meat. Try this way of eating kimchi. Take a little bit of meat, top it up with hot kimchi, pop it in your mouth, and cool yourself down with a mouth full of bland rice. Do not eat it by itself. You can also try kimchi sandwiches, by layering some bread with meat, kimchi, green lettuce, butter, cheese, tomatoes and cucumber. Talk about subs!

Also, try kimchi omelette, where you are going to eat eggs with chopped onions, spices and seasonings, and made piquant with kimchi.

Traditional Radish Stuffed Bread-Mooli Parantha

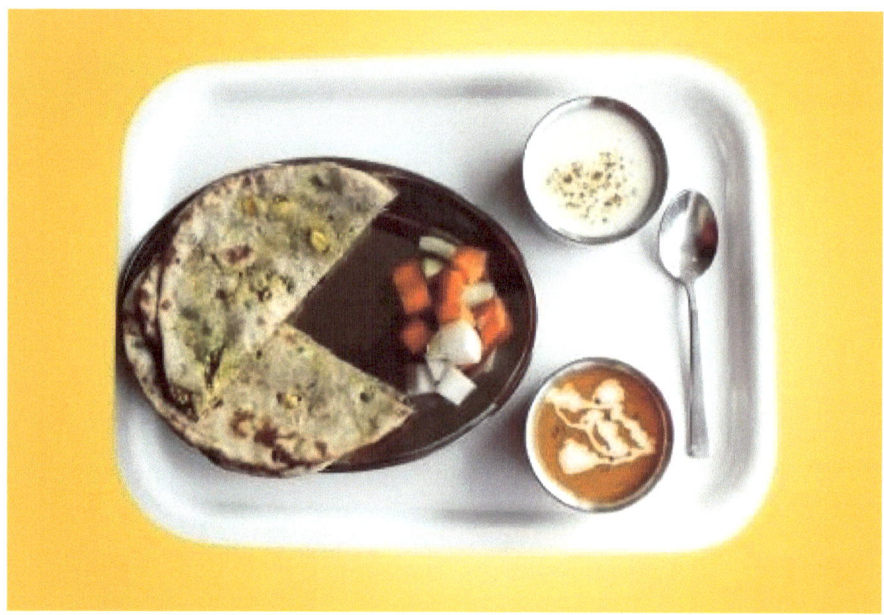

This stuffed bread has been served with yogurt with some chopped onions- Raitha- and spiced with black salt and pepper. The other dish with cream on it looks to be some masala gravy with cream.

North Indians love stuffing of their breads –roti, with anything like potatoes, but radishes come a close second.

This is the traditional recipe for stuffed bread, also known as parantha which differs from the basic Indian roti, because it is fried on a griddle pan with desi ghee, after it has been folded a number of times.

My grandmother used to make stuffed potato paranthas every Sunday, but it was only when I came to North India in my 30s, that I got to know all about this traditional culture which demanded radish paranthas every day made up of pure desi ghee and with a buttermilk accompaniment.

This is a breakfast dish of all the north Indian farmers out there, ready to go for a hard day's work on their land. When I was first confronted with it, I was put off with the completely raw smell of frying radish and frying desi ghee, both of them are very powerful and aromatic. And I asked my rustic hostess what she thought about the smell. She smiled and said that everybody who has had this breakfast, is going to smell the same, so nobody bothers!

Talk about being practical.

The basic bread is going to be made up of 250 g of whole wheat flour
Salt 1 teaspoon
4 tablespoons full of desi ghee
¾ cup water.

Mix them all together to make a firm dough. Cover with a cloth and place in a warm place for half an hour, while you gather together the rest of the stuffing mixture.

The stuffing mixture is going to consist of 250 g grated radishes, one media money in, 1 inch piece of fresh ginger, ¾ teaspoon roasted and powdered cumin seed, pepper and salt to taste, and two green chilies. You can add as many spices as you wish to make the spicy bread. I normally add some bishops weed to give it an even more tangy taste.

Mash the radishes together with salt. Mix in the onion, ginger and chilies together Now heat the ghee in a skillet, add all these mixed ingredients and fry them slightly until the onions are slightly cooked. Now add the radishes along with salt, pepper, cumin seed, and any other spices you wish. Cook on low heat for a few minutes and allow to cool.

Now make a ball of the dough and flatten with the palm of your hand. Roll the ball with your rolling pin, apply a little bit of desi ghee, add some of the stuffing, and then fold in half. Now you have a stuffed semicircle. Fold again until you have a square. This is the basis of the parantha, which is now going to be rolled out and flattened with your rolling pin.

Remember, too much of the stuffing is going to come out of the corners, when you apply the rolling pin again to the square.

Heat your griddle pan, apply a little bit of Desi ghee to the surface of the griddle, and place your bread on it. Allow to fry on low heat for about half a minute, while applying some Desi ghee on the other surface. When the frying surfaces, lightly cooked, turn it over. You are going to see light Brown spots, which shows that yes, the bread has been cooked. All the while, the other surface is being fried. You may want to turn it a couple more times until it is completely crisp and both the sides are delicious Golden Brown.

Serve piping hot with yogurt in which onions have been chopped, garnished with mint and salt and pepper.

These are supposedly said not to keep very well, but I preserved them by placing them when still steaming, in a cloth, to preserve the steam, and then placed them straight in a plastic bag right into the freezer. Whenever you want to eat it, you just place the **unfrosted** parantha in the microwave, and there you are with this fresh, crisp, and delicious bread.

This reminds me of an old amusing story of soldiers and officers serving at high altitudes, especially in Leh- Ladakh about 15 years ago. [This procedure is still practiced and very much in use today!]

Any officer whether he belonged to the Army or the Air Force posted in that area and going home on annual leave was/is immediately given an order by all of his colleagues to get homemade *aloo* – potato – or *mooli* – radish – paranthas for the whole unit. Otherwise, he need not come back to the unit/base on pain of immediate justified pesticide!

Naturally, these paranthas are to be made up of Desi ghee; nothing less will do for these hard-working gourmands.

Those paranthas were/are then lovingly buried in the ice, and dug up when needed by the hungry officers and men. These places were marked with red markers, so that people got to know exactly where to dig when they were feeling nostalgic and wanted some homemade food cooked by a mother's, wife's or a sister's caring hands.

Now one fine day, one young, healthy, hearty, and naturally always hungry Flying Officer decided to keep the knowledge of all those buried treasures to himself. Therefore, he changed the positions of all the markers.

When my brother and his friends decided on some fresh home made paranthas, made by yours truly, they went to the markers and found absolutely nothing.

Consternation all around!

Where were those homemade delicacies, to be eaten with mango pickles and yogurt and washed down with any not so soft drink in the Mess?

More consternation when the Flying Officer went to the place where he thought those paranthas were buried, and found out that he had forgotten the locations. His final fate at the hands of his friends, seniors and fellow colleagues is not documented.

But his friends say that they punished him by making him dig in the cold, cold, snow, all during his leisure time, and in all Weathers. But Alas, No joy!

As that is a high-altitude area, where the snow never melts, there are three packets of 24 paranthas each, buried deep in the snow and nobody knows where they are. One caring sister made them for the whole unit consisting of her then bachelor brother and his young equally hungry youthful friends, colleagues and seniors. And as they are preserved in the snow and steam frozen, they were still be as tasty today, as they would be fresh off the griddle.

So now, how do you make Desi ghee?

If you buy it in the market, it is exorbitantly priced, especially when you do not know that you are buying the real thing. Nowadays, you may find something in the market, pretending to be this concentrated clarified butter, but is actually a mixture of vegetable oils and some desi ghee for the flavor. So if you have a source where you can get lots of fresh and pure unsalted butter, you can make it right at home.

Desi ghee is clarified butter, which is extremely concentrated and a very powerful healing agent. It is normally used in the making up of herbal medicines, because it is made of pure creamy milk butter. It is also used in making beauty creams, potions, lotions and other skin ointments.

It has a powerful aroma, and that is why only just a spoonful is added to fry meats. It is going to float on the surface of the meat dish, after it has been cooked, so you need to stir the gravy before serving. Also, the food is not going to taste greasy, even though it looks like it has been swimming in fat.

Desi ghee is pure butter, which is heated to reduce the butter of all the impurities as well as moisture. This concentrated butter is normally used in Eastern cuisine, for searing meat, sautéing and frying food, because they offer its higher burning point. You make this at home by taking 2 pounds of best unsalted butter and melting it in a heavy bottomed pan. Allow the butter to liquefy on low heat for about 40 minutes. Maintain this simmering point, until all of the moisture in the butter has evaporated. The impurities are going to sink to the bottom of the pan. Remember to keep stirring the butter, so that it does not burn.

Pour off the clear butter and strain it through several thicknesses of muslin cloth. This butter is going to last for about a year, if it is placed in a cool and dry place. This butter is exorbitantly expensive. So in the East, people with easy access to plenty fresh milk make it right in their kitchens for crisp delicious frying results, and adding that taste of pure butter to all their dishes.

Radishes to Cure

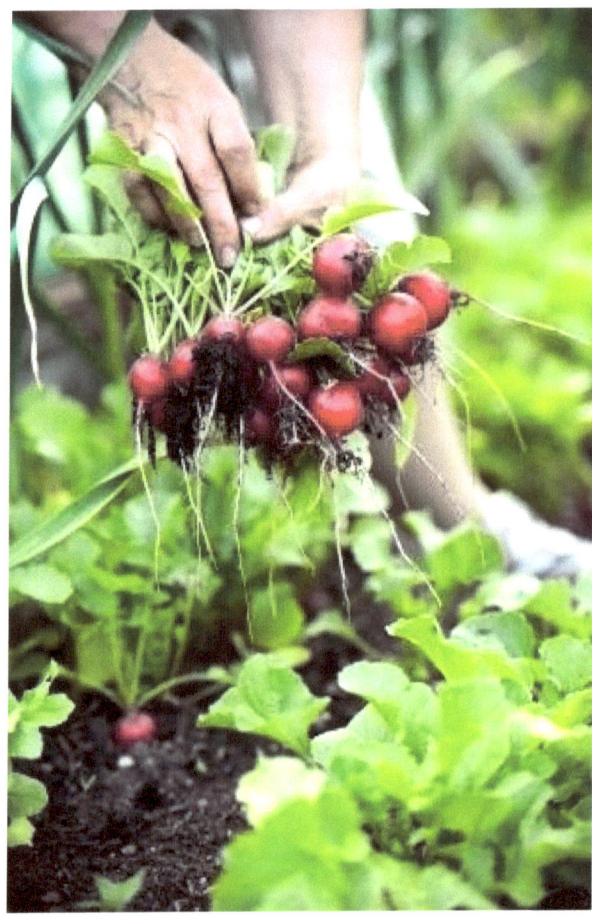

An ancient told me the secret of his good health and longevity. He got rid of anybody in short problems, right at the very beginning by eating at least one radish every day. For breakfast he had one whole unskinned radish   with lemons, and for lunch, he had radish salad, along with tomatoes, and carrots, especially in the winters. This cured potential gastric problems, related to bile as well as acidic problems in the digestive system. Also, it got rid of any parasites in the stomach, especially when he drank one teaspoonful of lemon juice, with a little bit of rock salt twice a day for two days when he thought that his appetite was failing and the parasites had had time to grow in his intestines.

I began to do that even though I do not suffer from digestive problems. But this is a good way to get some carrots and tomatoes into my vegetable – avoiding – system.

Get Rid of Skin Diseases with Radishes

Radish juice is excellent for getting rid of skin diseases. This is an excellent blood purifier and that is why it is given to children in the summer as a boiled vegetable so that they do not suffer from boils, skin infections or other "impure blood" related problems.

Remember that if you are using radish to purify your blood, do not add any salt to it. This salt is going to prevent the curing of skin diseases. Also try applying freshly grated radishes to a boil or an infected area on your skin to see how fast it is cured.

Eczema Cure

I normally recommend turpentine for people suffering from eczema, but you can also try crushing the seeds of radish, with some lemon juice. Now heat this mixture in your spoon a bit and apply directly on to the eczema spot. Or you may just want to make a paste of dried radish leaves with water and apply it on the affected area. Try not to scratch it, because that is going to spread the infection. If you are using the dry leaves cure, repeat this 2 to 3 times a day until your skin reaches its normal smooth, healthy state.

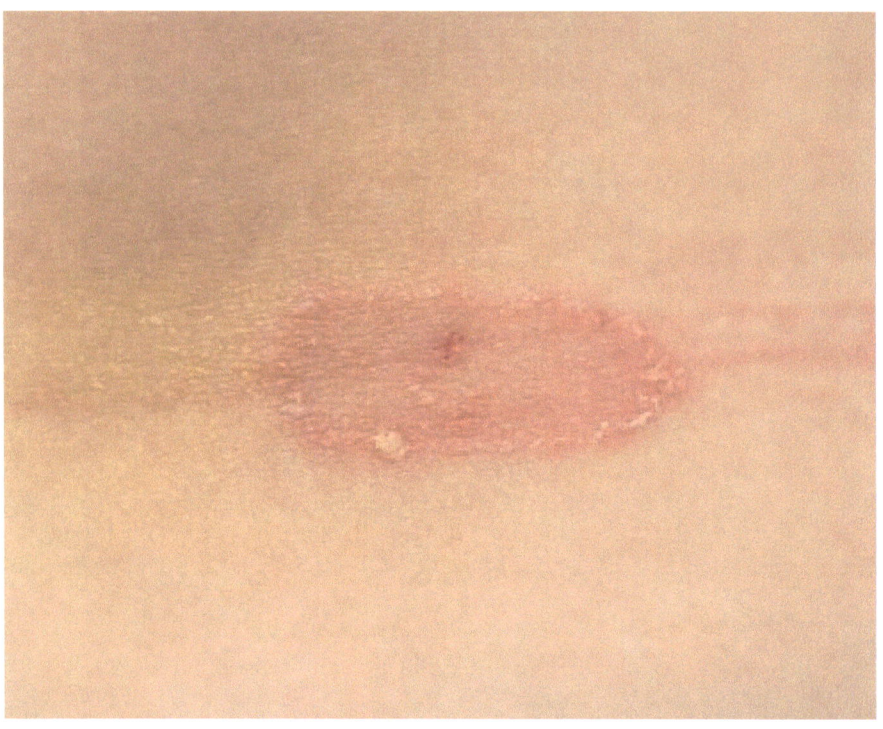

You will never suffer from eczema again if you have radishes around.

Blemishes on Your Skin?

Try this remedy. Grind some radish seeds with water and apply the paste all over the blemishes, until they disappear. This is also a good way in which you can get rid of wrinkles.

The best remedy for these blemishes are 2 tablespoons full of fresh radish juice, raw radish leaves and radishes in salads. Thanks to the sulfur and potassium content in the radishes, your skin is going to get its natural beautiful glow again. This remedy, however, is going to take 20 – 25 days to show its full curative potential and power. The fresh leaves of the radish also stop your skin from itching.

If you find your scalp itching and you think that you are suffering from dandruff, why not try washing the scalp with radish juice? This is going to stink, but it is guaranteed effective.

Appetite Enhancer

Just imagine that you are feeling hungry, but do not wish to eat anything. This normally happens when people are stressed out and they do not want to take time out to eat something nutritious. Under such circumstances and conditions, their bodies going to be deprived of all the essential nutrients which are necessary to keep you fit and fine.

So try this appetite enhancer right now. Slice the middle of a radish without dividing it into two. Now fill up that cut with a mixture of lemon juice, and rock salt. Eat with mint chutney. And then see your appetite coming back with a roar.

This is also the **traditional ulcer cure**, where you are going to eat transversely cut radishes and filled with lemon juice, without salt and without the mint chutney. Also, remember to eat the raw fresh young leaves of the radish along with the lemon – radish.

This helps curing the intestinal linings, and preventing the acidic content of the stomach from harming them, and creating even more ulcers.

People suffering from ulcers need to avoid, rich and fatty foods. Also, they have to cut down on sour and spicy foods. Such foods increase the acidic content of the stomach, and aggravate the ulcers.

Traditional appetizing and digestive Mint Chutney

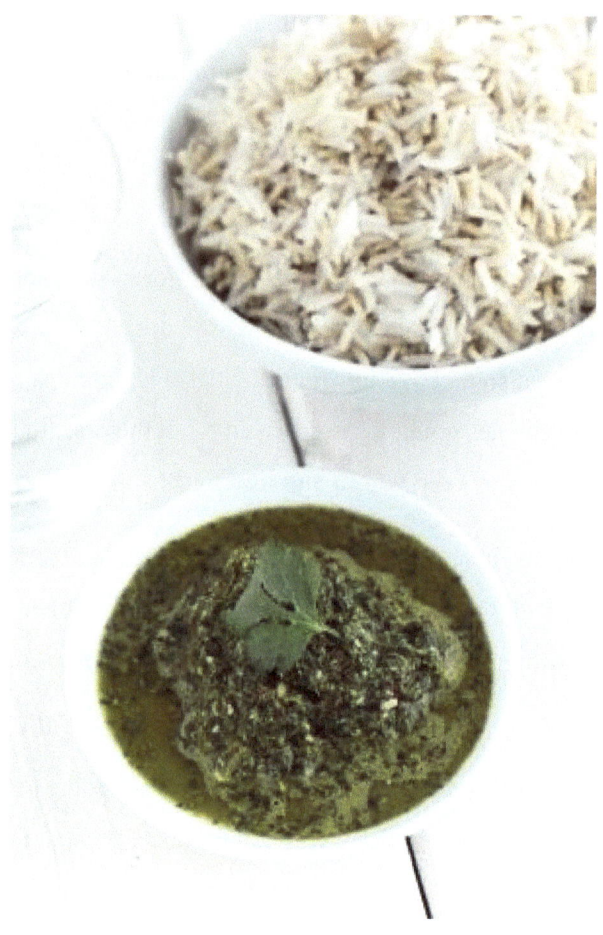

This is made fresh every morning in summer in eastern kitchens, to be given to the family with their meals. This is going to cool down the system, in preparation for the hot summer's day.

Try eating the stuffed bread given above, with this chutney. Seriously yummy.

¼ Pound fresh mint leaves, washed and dried

One medium-sized onion

Juice of 1 ½ limes

4 tablespoons minced parsley and coriander(cilantro)

Half a teaspoonful of red chillies for hot chutney, a pinch for really mild chutney

1 teaspoon full rock salt

¼ Teaspoon black salt.

Pepper to taste

Two teaspoons full honey.

I normally use mint leaves, but you may want to put in some tender stalks. Mix the onion in the blender with a little bit of lime juice. Then add the mint, parsley, etc., and the remaining lime juice. Blend for 10 seconds, and then add all the spices and seasonings. Blend and grind well. This is best served chilled.

This chutney is a little liquefied because of the lemon. Use the dry chutney to make an amazing sandwich spread.

You can also spread on buttered whole-wheat bread, with a little bit of grated cheese and mayonnaise. This is then sprinkled with garlic salt, rock salt and black pepper. You may want to put some tomatoes, and some green lettuce to make a sandwich hamburger.

In the same manner, you can also spread mint chutney on roasted hamburgers, before stuffing with pieces of cheese and tomatoes between sesame whole-wheat hamburger buns and enjoying.

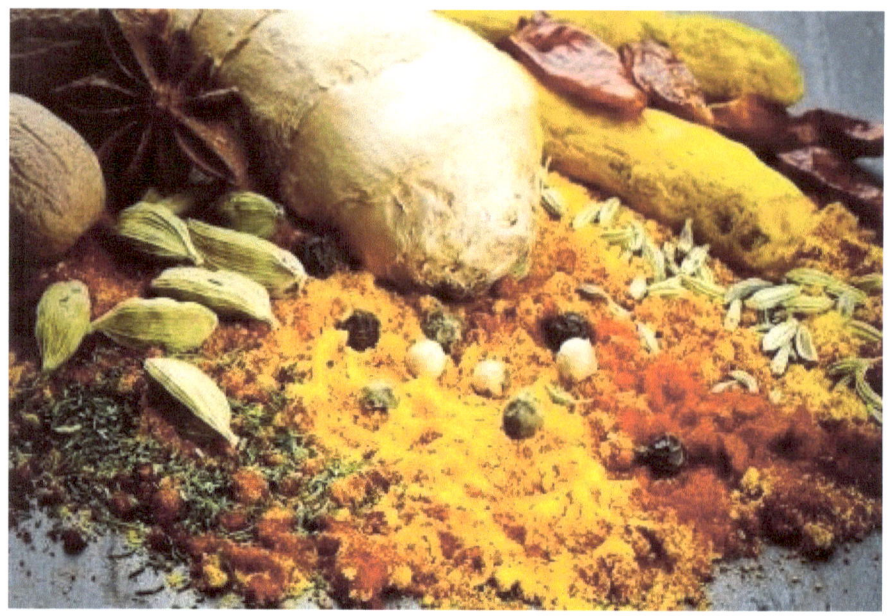

Indian street food just cannot do without mint chutney accompanied with chopped tomatoes, radishes, onions, yogurt, tamarind chutney, and spicy mint- water.

People suffering from colon problems, ulcers and digestive problems are recommended **not to eat radishes on its own or in a raw form. The ulcer remedy is going to be given to you further on.** These problems are going to be aggravated due to the added radish intake. Even though since ancient times, the leaves of the radishes considered to be the best way in which the body can get rid of the toxins, you should only eat them if you have a healthy digestive system and do not suffer from stomach related digestive ailments.

Tummy ache

However, you can get rid of tummy ache by drinking one teaspoonful of radish juice with a pinch of rock salt.

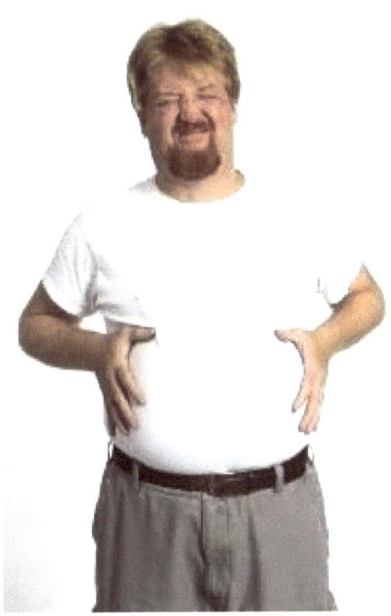

A Tablespoon full of radish juice with lemon juice and some rock salt can help prevent tummy problems brought about by overeating.

Dropsy

This was a remedy which I saw being used to cure a person of dropsy. Under such circumstances, the patient starts retaining water in his tummy area. And that water retention moves from side to side, as he changes sides, when lying down.

Radishes have been proven to cure dropsy since ancient times.

Try this proven remedy right now. Take 10 g of radish juice and add 6 teaspoons of ginger juice to this mixture. Now give the patient 1 tablespoon of this mixture, three times a day. You are going to see all that retained water being removed from the body, within 4 to 5 days.

Make sure that the patient suffering from dropsy does not eat anything salty, while undertaking this cure. Salt retains water in the body.

I have never suffered from dropsy, but I do know that if there is some water retention in my body, it is because of an increased salt intake. 24 – 40 hours without salt and all those toxins go out of my system on the second – third day.

Flatulence Problems

Prevent flatulence and also cure it by eating a salad of some radish leaves along with sliced radishes, cucumbers, lemon juice and sprinkled with rock salt. Tasty to eat, and gets rid of any flatulence problems. Do not get rid of the radish skin or peel it, when you are making this salad.

Also, if somebody is suffering from chronic flatulence, grate a radish without peeling it. Now, drink the juice and reduce the intake of salt. In the same manner, eat unpeeled cucumbers and drink their juice. This is going to take a while to get rid of all the flatulence problems, but believe me, it works.

Radishes for Your Hair

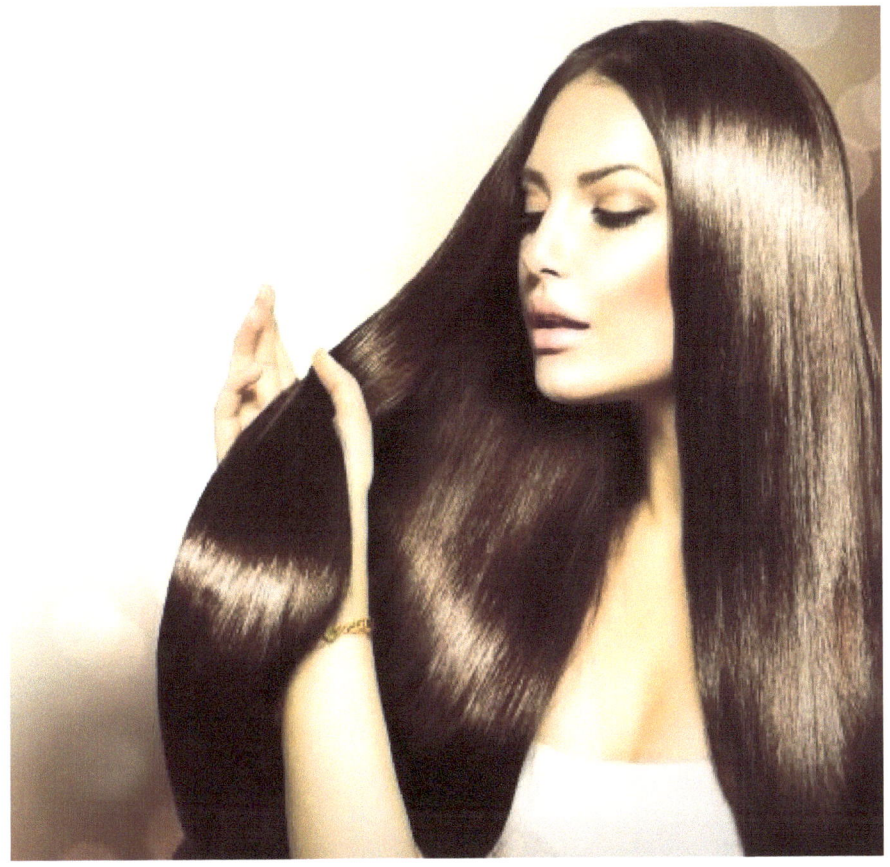

A diet rich in radishes can keep your hair healthy and shining

I did not know that radishes were excellent for encouraging your hair growth, but thanks to the silicon and phosphorous content in this vegetable, you can prevent yourself from growing bald due to hair loss.

Start eating unpeeled radishes and unpeeled cucumbers. Add wheat germs and germinated mung sprouts to your daily diet. Any raw vegetable or fruit you eat should have its peeling on, including citrus fruits. This is a good way to prevent any possible potential hair loss in the future.

Hair Growth

If you are genetically prone to white hair at a young age, thanks to your ancestors and your genes, it is impossible for you to darken your hair from the hair roots. Nevertheless, if you find yourself with an expected white hair, due to health reasons or any other external circumstances like the pollution in the atmosphere, add radishes, onions, tomatoes, cauliflowers and turnips to your diet. These are going to provide your body with all those essential ingredients and minerals necessary to encourage a healthy hair growth.

Dental Care

Radishes are excellent for tooth care.

Never suffer from toothache or shaking teeth ever again as long as you have radishes around.

Shaking Teeth

I was wondering about a reason why many villagers I knew did not suffer from teeth problems, even when they were in their 70s and 80s. They told me that they kept their teeth healthy by biting off pieces of radish and chewing it, every day. Also, anybody suffering from shaking teeth was immediately made to gargle with 50 mL of radish juice in one glass of warm water first thing every morning for 20 to 25 days. This water was also swished around the teeth before spitting out.

Do this for 10 minutes, so that all the affected areas are bathed in radish juice. After that, drink 2 tablespoons of fresh radish juice.

Once your teeth start getting healed, keep them healthy by eating radishes every day. Bite, chew, and allow your teeth to get plenty of exercise with fresh radishes.

This was supposed to be the best way in which they managed to keep their teeth shining, healthy, and firm and did not suffer from dental problems.

Pyorrhea Cure

Try this out, if you find your dental bills escalating as you grow older. Do not try chewing radishes, if you have shaking teeth. Instead, apply the pulp of a fresh radish   on the surface of those affected teeth and on the gums. This also prevents and cures pyorrhea.

Toothache

If you have a painful tooth, do not chew on a radish, because, well, your tooth is playing merry pranks with your nerves. Instead, make a pulp of the radish, add the juice of one lemon to it and place it under the painful tooth. Now masticate the pulp slowly until all the juice reaches the paining and infected area.

I also tried the warm water radish juice fomentation remedy of taking a mouthful of this warm liquid and allowing the warmth to seep around the affected area and bring it relief. It worked.

Insomnia Remedy

I noticed that I slept better at night, if I ate a salad made up of onions and radishes with dinner. When I asked my herbalist friend, if that particular diet had something to do to cure my state of chronic insomnia, he said that yes, it was helpful and that I could try adding one raw radish to my lunch and then see how I slept like the proverbial top.

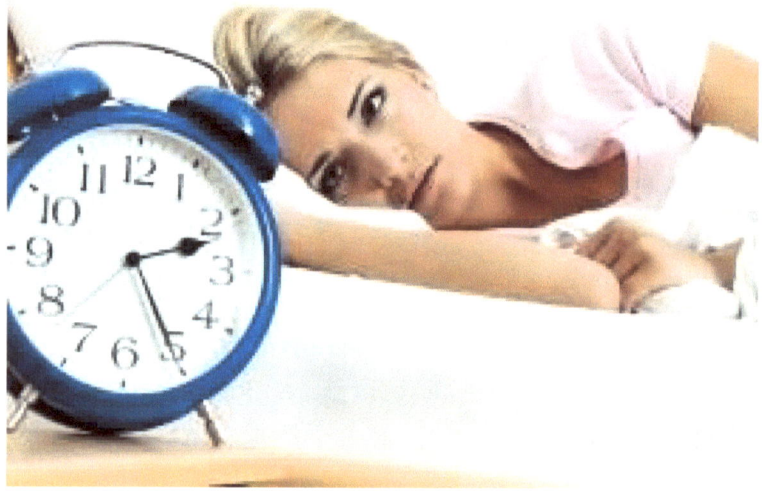

No more sleepless nights when you have radish juice at hand.

Conclusion

This book just gives you some of the natural remedies and recipes, coming down from ancient times in which radishes have been utilized for the benefit of mankind. The natural remedies given here are time-tested, and for common ailments, because after all, one would rather go to a doctor and get expensive chemical-based drugs, than trying out something, which has been in use for millenniums.

Nevertheless, the importance of radishes in alternative medicine is something which can definitely not be overlooked. Korean, Chinese and other Eastern and Ancient cuisine was based on the fact that the cooks knew all about the necessary minerals and elements, which were needed by the body to function properly. That is why they made sure that the dishes that were prepared had the perfect balance of all the essential nutrients in one tasty dish. This is the principle on which ancient and traditional cuisine worked, and it is still being practiced to this day.

The magic series brought to you thus introduces the good things of a plant, herb, spice, flower or vegetable, and encourages you to look at the natural way in which to keep healthy.

Nature has provided you with all this magnificent bounty, so that you can take full advantage of her munificence. The ancients have provided you with the knowledge, which you just need to understand and utilize. And so it is in your hands to make sure that your life is full of good health and energy. The natural way is the simplest way in which you can follow the path of living, set down by the ancients so successfully, easily, absolutely and effectively.

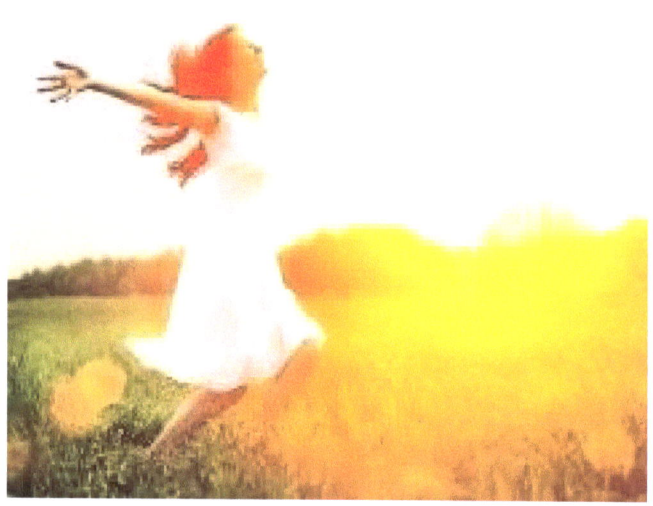

Live long and prosper the natural way!

Author Bio

Dueep Jyot Singh is a Management and IT Professional who managed to gather Postgraduate qualifications in Management and English and Degrees in Science, French and Education while pursuing different enjoyable career options like being an hospital administrator, IT,SEO and HRD Database Manager/ trainer, movie scriptwriter, theatre artiste and public speaker, lecturer in French, Marketing and Advertising, ex-Editor of Hearts On Fire (now known as Solctice) Books Missouri USA, advice columnist and cartoonist, publisher and Aviation School trainer, ex- moderator on Medico.in, banker, student councilor ,travelogue writer … among other things! One fine morning, she decided that she had enough of killing herself by Degrees and went back to her first love -- writing. It's more enjoyable! She already has 48 published academic and 14 fiction- in- different- genre books under her belt.

When she is not designing websites or making Graphic design illustrations for clients …including R.L. Stevenson, O.Henry, Dornford Yates, Maurice Walsh, C.N.Williamson, Sapper, Bartimeus and the crown of her collection-Dickens "The Old Curiosity Shop," and so on… Just call her "Renaissance Woman" - collecting herbal remedies, acting like Universal Helping Hand/Agony Aunt, or escaping to her dear mountains for a bit of exploring, collecting herbs and plants, and trekking.

Check out some of the other JD-Biz Publishing books

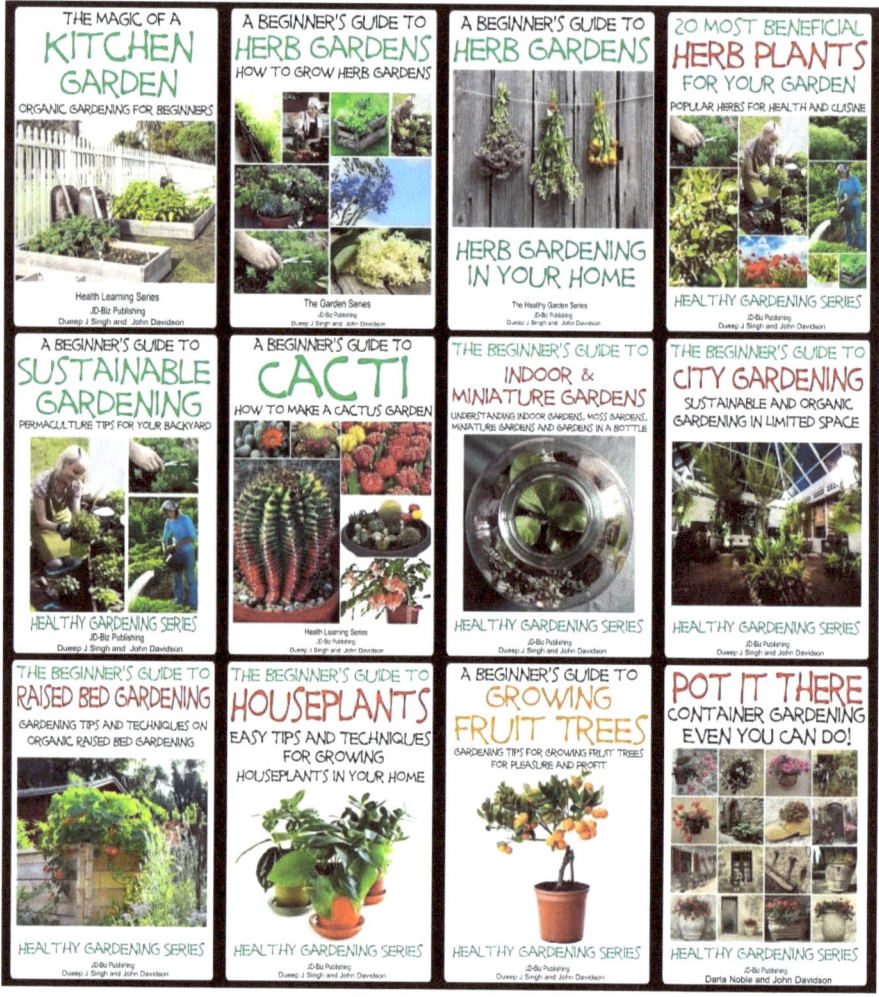

Download Free Books!

http://MendonCottageBooks.com

Health Learning Series

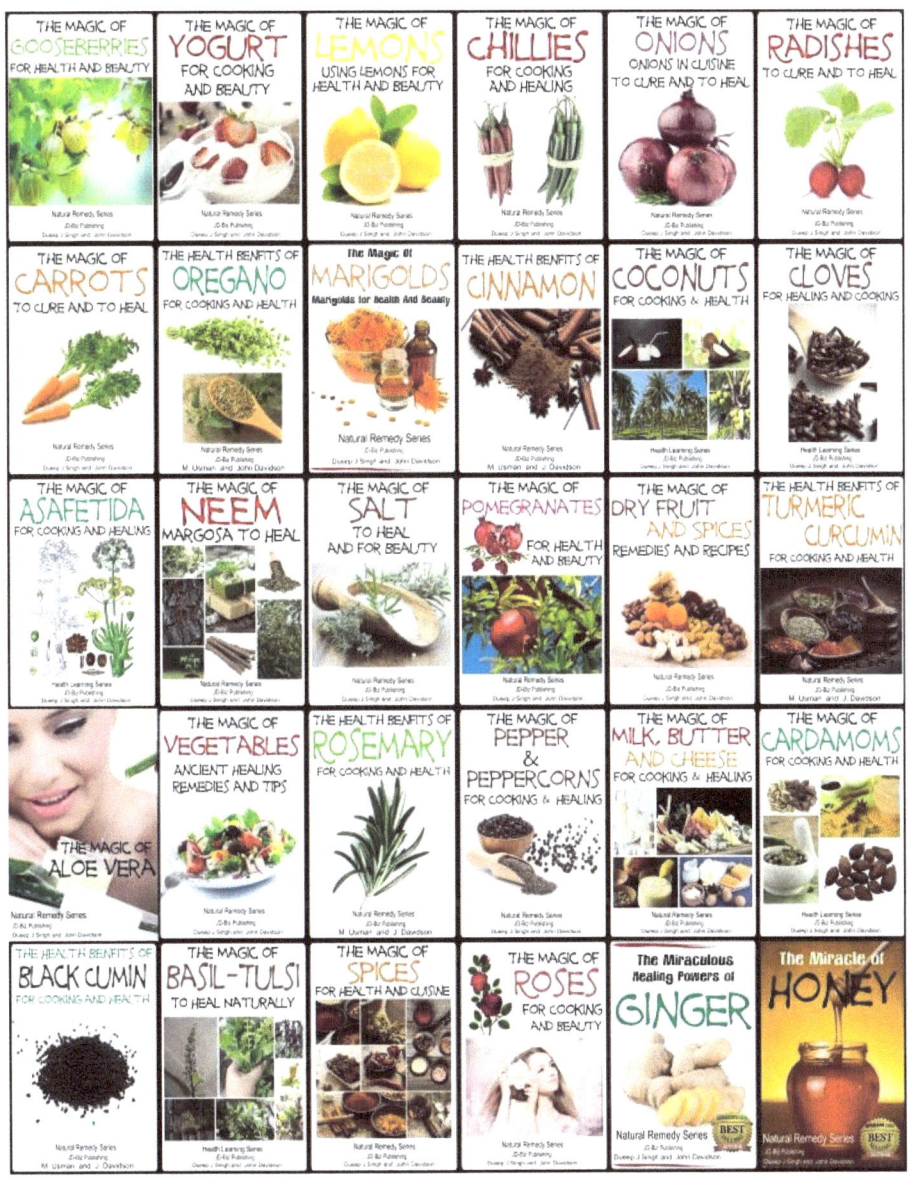

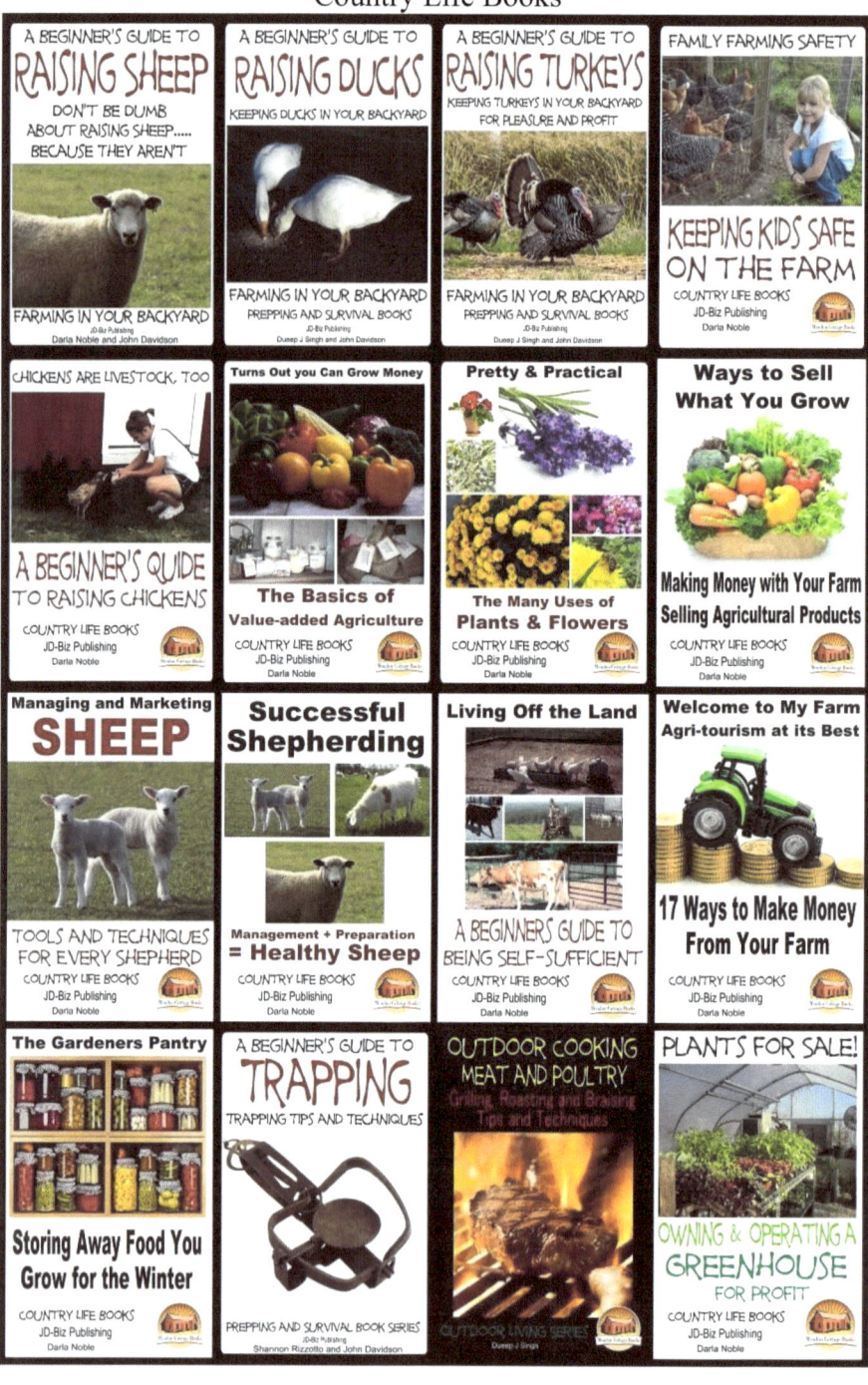

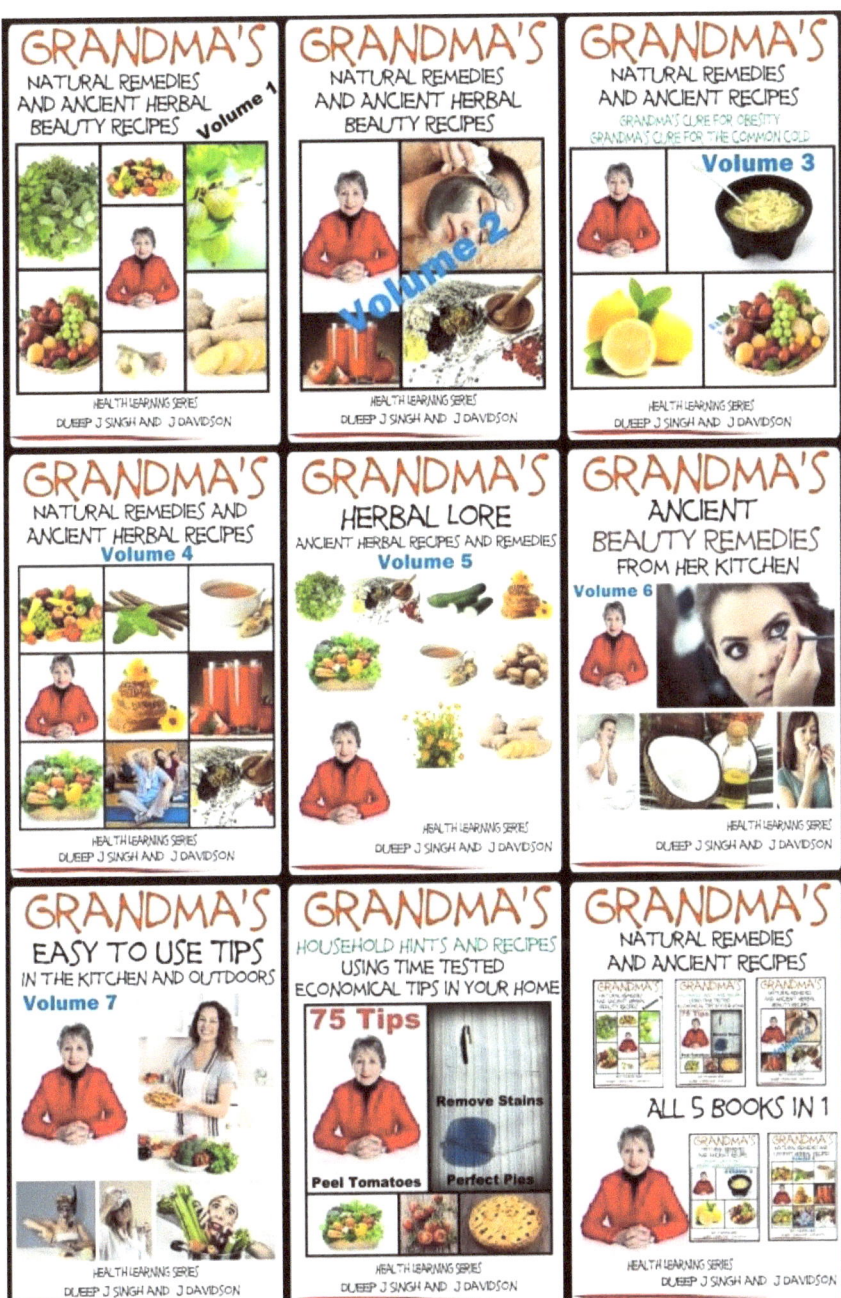

Health Learning Series

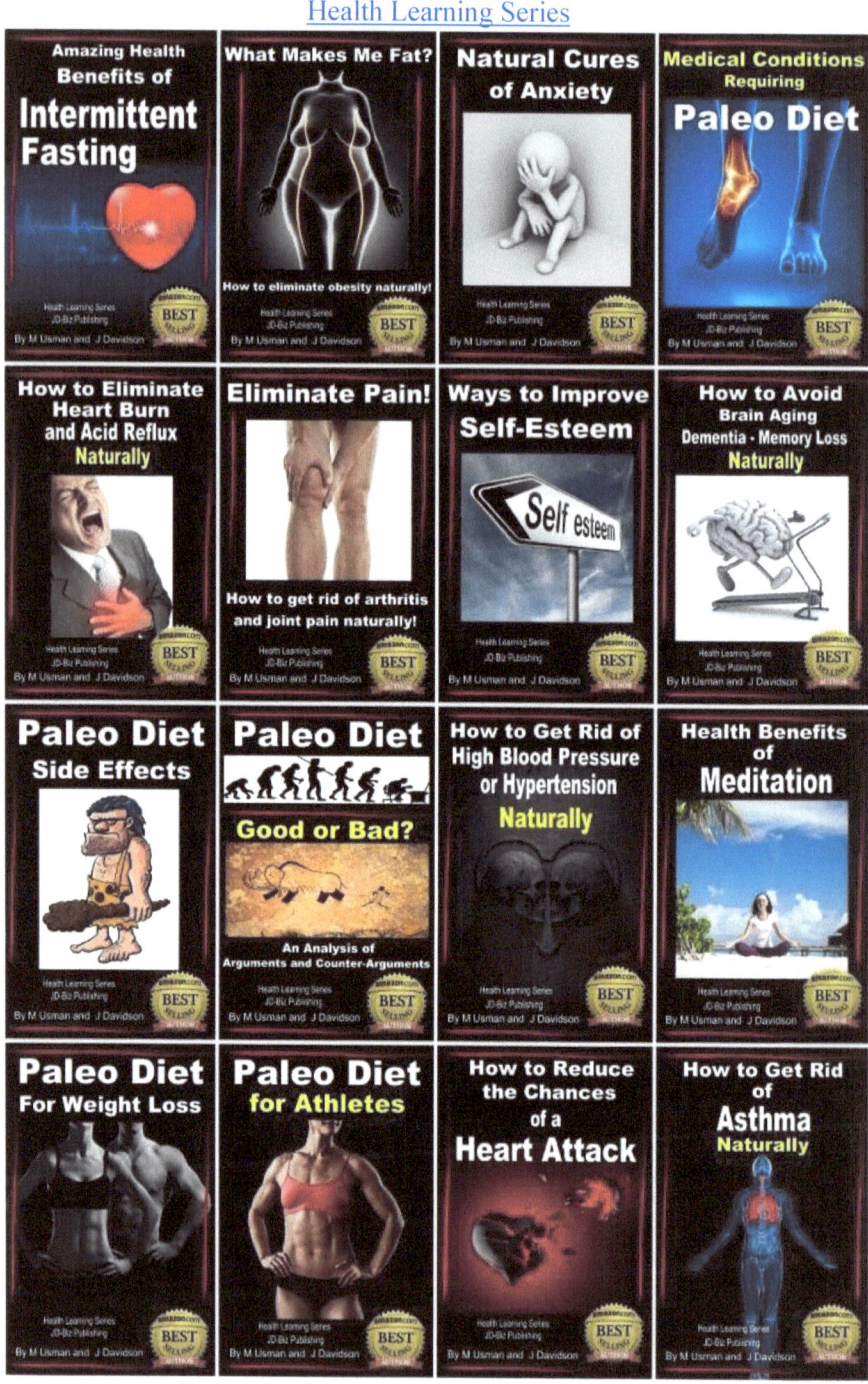

Amazing Animal Book Series

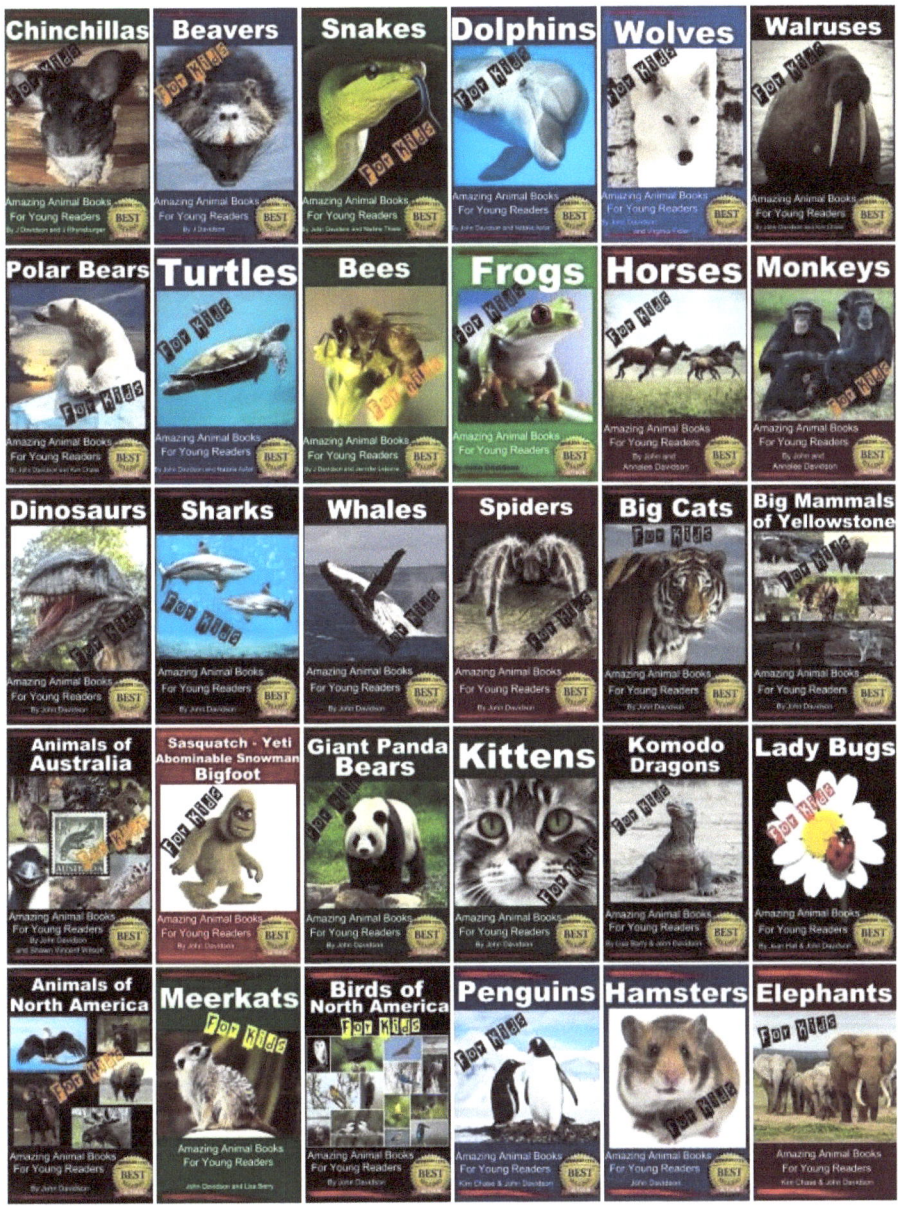

Learn To Draw Series

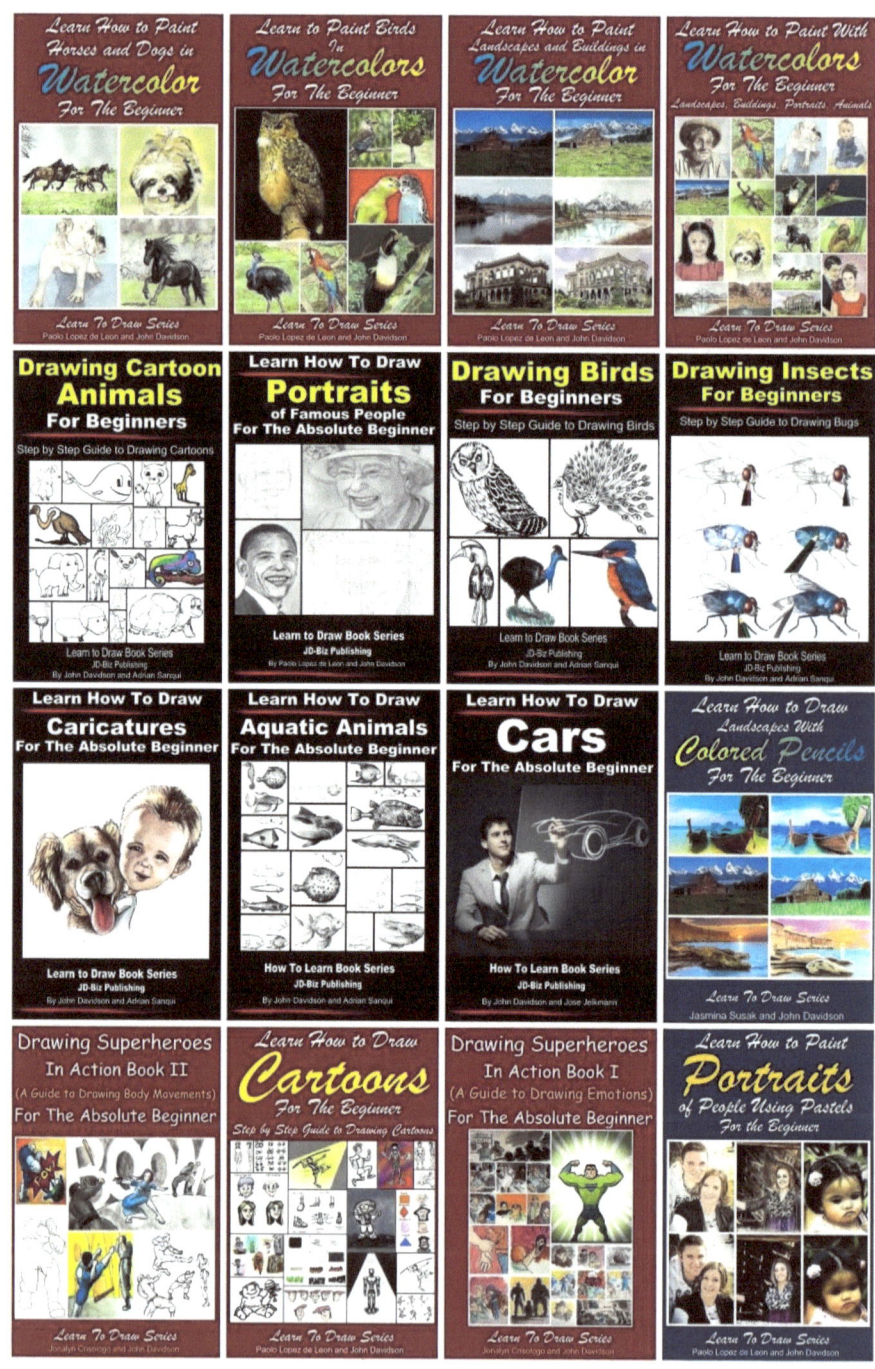

How to Build and Plan Books

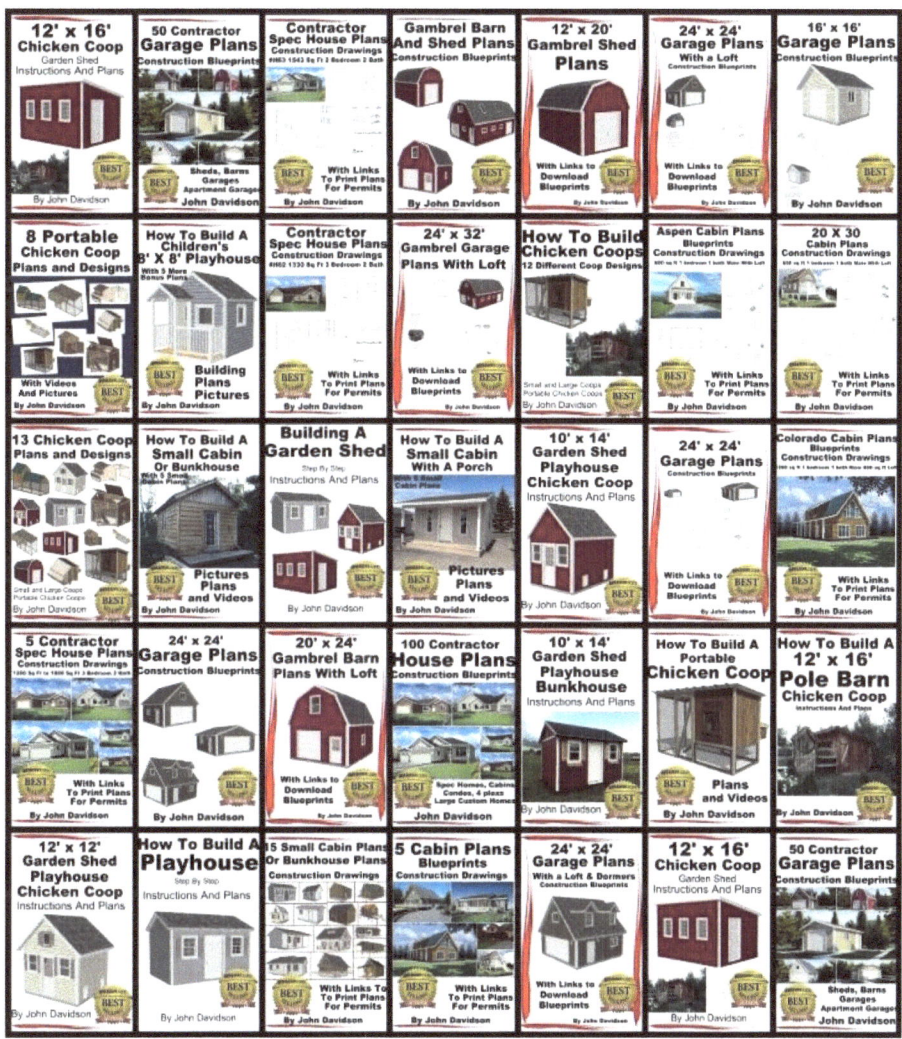

Entrepreneur Book Series

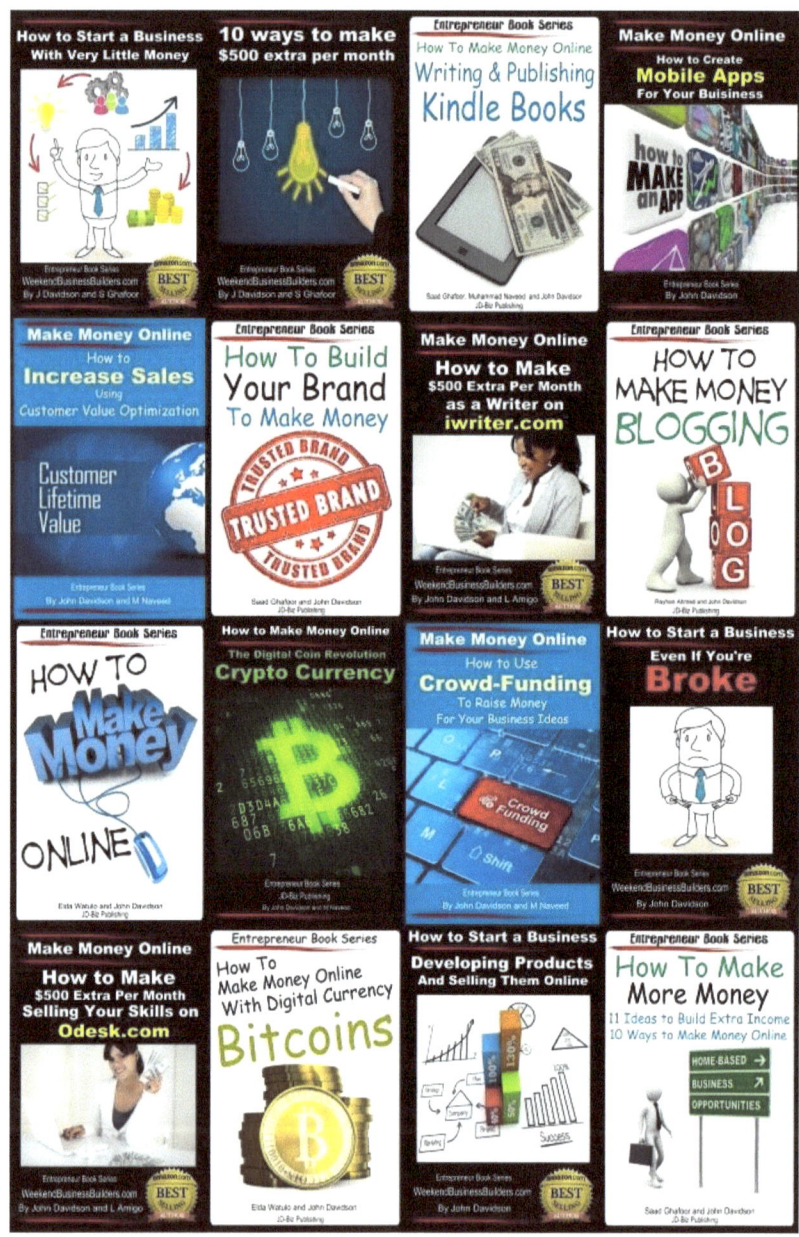

Our books are available at

1. Amazon.com

2. Barnes and Noble

3. Itunes

4. Kobo

5. Smashwords

6. Google Play Books

Download Free Books!

http://MendonCottageBooks.com

Publisher

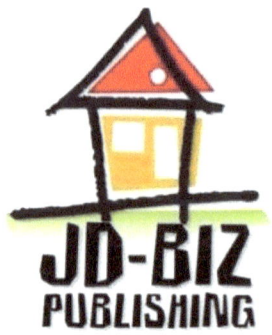

JD-Biz Corp

P O Box 374

Mendon, Utah 84325

http://www.jd-biz.com/

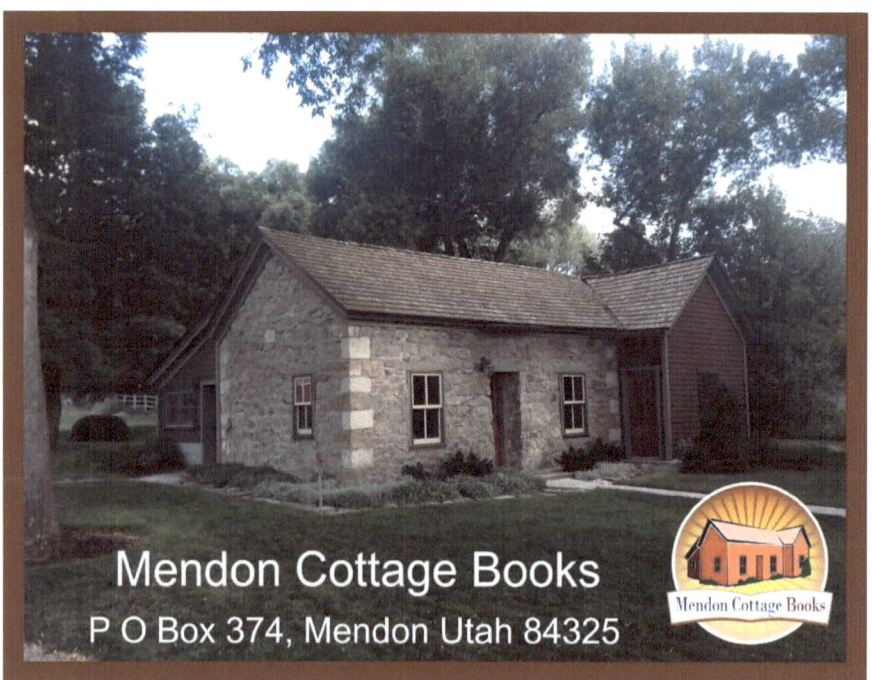